T H E
daniel fast
WORKBOOK

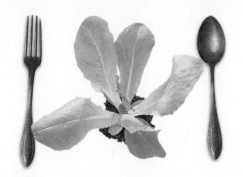

THE
daniel
fast

WORKBOOK

susan gregory

TYNDALE™
MOMENTUM

An Imprint of
Tyndale House Publishers, Inc.

Visit Tyndale online at www.tyndale.com.

Visit Tyndale Momentum online at www.tyndalemomentum.com.

Visit the author's website at www.daniel-fast.com.

TYNDALE is a registered trademark of Tyndale House Publishers, Inc. *Tyndale Momentum* and the Tyndale Momentum logo are trademarks of Tyndale House Publishers, Inc. Tyndale Momentum is an imprint of Tyndale House Publishers, Inc.

The Daniel Fast Workbook: A 5-Week Guide for Individuals, Groups, and Churches

ISBN 978-1-4143-8790-1 Softcover

Printed in the United States of America

19   18   17   16   15   14   13
7   6   5   4   3   2

Dedication

....

I DEDICATE THIS BOOK to the worldwide Daniel Fast community who came together on *The Daniel Fast* blog and website. You have led me to deep and powerful truths about our Kingdom of God life as I researched answers to your questions and pondered your comments. You have encouraged me with your kind letters and messages of support. You have joined me with your virtual presence and financial support as we ministered to the men, women, and children in southern Africa. And you have taken my hand as we work together to let others know about the precious and powerful gifts available to the children of God through prayer and fasting.

I am honored to be a member of this community with you. Thank you, dear friends. While I can't list your individual names here, please know that I am truly grateful to you for making this book possible . . . I dedicate it to you. May the peace of Christ continue to overtake every part of your lives.

Table of Contents

Before You Begin

THE DANIEL FAST includes a very healthy eating plan. However, please allow the Great Physician to work hand in hand with your earthly physician. Any time you make a significant change to your diet and exercise routines, it's a good idea to check with your health professional for his or her input.

Fasting should never harm the body. If you have special dietary needs—if you are pregnant or nursing, if you have a chronic illness such as cancer or diabetes, if you are a young person who is still growing or an athlete who expends more than typical amounts of energy on a regular basis—contact your health professional and modify the Daniel Fast eating plan in a way that is appropriate for your unique situation.

Welcome to the Daniel Fast

IF YOU ARE preparing to embark on the Daniel Fast—either individually or as part of a group—you are about to enter a life-changing spiritual adventure!

In the Old Testament book of Daniel, we learn that the young prophet and his companions entered a partial fast (restricting food for a spiritual purpose) so they could remain true to their God—instead of eating meat and wine that had been dedicated to the Babylonian false gods. Fashioned on Daniel's experiences recorded in Daniel 1 and 10, the Daniel Fast is a partial fast in which some foods are restricted, creating an eating plan similar to a vegan diet (completely plant-based with no animal products).

The purpose of the fast is to abstain from certain foods for a fixed period of time in order to focus our attention more deliberately on our relationship with God and to allow God to speak to us about specific issues in our lives. As we intentionally limit what we eat and bring our physical appetites under control, God invites us to feast on His abundant strength and provision.

After communicating with thousands of men, women, and teens about the Daniel Fast, I've discovered that what people want most are instructions. They don't just want to know *about* fasting; they also want to know *how to fast*. That's why I wrote the book *The Daniel Fast* and have dedicated myself to sharing its message through my website and blog (www.daniel-fast.com).

But I've also discovered that people need *purpose* and *encouragement* during a fast, which is what prompted me to create this workbook. *Purpose* enables us to stay faithful to the guiding motives and principles of our fast. This book is written with that key goal in mind: helping you establish your purpose and keep it at the forefront of your mind and heart. *Encouragement* is necessary because changing our habits can be daunting, even when we have a higher purpose in mind. It's important for you to know you're not alone in the journey.

My goal for *The Daniel Fast Workbook* is to walk with you with purpose and encouragement through the *actual fasting experience*, covering a five-week period: one week of preparation, three weeks (twenty-one days) of fasting, and a concluding week of reflection and celebration. You can use this workbook as a personal study guide if you are doing the fast on your own, or you can use it in a group setting with your church or small group.

No matter how you do it, fasting will always be a solitary journey to some degree. After all, *only you* can decide for yourself to give up certain foods for a season as a spiritual exercise. And you must come to that decision on your own. But once you have decided to fast, it can be helpful to join your efforts with the efforts of others, to share insights and encourage one another along the way. That's what I want to do for you in *The Daniel Fast Workbook* and what I hope you will do for each other if you are fasting with a group.

Psalm 34:1-10 is a passage from God's Word on which to anchor your decision to participate in the Daniel Fast. I encourage you to meditate on this psalm while you prepare for the fast.

I will praise the Lord at all times.
　　I will constantly speak his praises.
I will boast only in the Lord;
　　let all who are helpless take heart.
Come, let us tell of the Lord's greatness;
　　let us exalt his name together.

I prayed to the Lord, and he answered me.
　　He freed me from all my fears.
Those who look to him for help will be radiant with joy;
　　no shadow of shame will darken their faces.
In my desperation I prayed, and the Lord listened;
　　he saved me from all my troubles.
For the angel of the Lord is a guard;
　　he surrounds and defends all who fear him.

Taste and see that the Lord is good.
　　Oh, the joys of those who take refuge in him!
Fear the Lord, you his godly people,
　　for those who fear him will have all they need.
Even strong young lions sometimes go hungry,
　　but those who trust in the Lord will lack no good thing.

As you read these words, I hope you sense a stirring of great anticipation and excitement. You are about to embark on a spiritual encounter that will open doors of understanding, growth, and faith like you have never known before.

Susan Gregory

How to Use This Workbook

....

THE FIVE-WEEK STUDY plan outlined in this workbook is designed for both groups and individuals. Though it's structured around a twenty-one-day fast, feel free to adjust for a shorter or longer time of fasting as it suits your needs.

In addition to this guide and your Bible, you will want my book *The Daniel Fast*, which is the basis for the reading plan that follows. It includes the practical information you will need regarding what foods are allowed on the fast, as well as dozens of recipes, meal plans, and a twenty-one-day devotional. I encourage you to read *The Daniel Fast* in its entirety as part of your preparation for the fast, and then review the recommended content each week to dig deeper into your fasting experience. (Others may prefer to read the book for the first time in week-by-week installments *during* the fast. This reading plan is adaptable for either approach.)

Because I have designed *The Daniel Fast Workbook* to mirror the questions and experiences you'll be having as you fast, you'll see that it is not a simple, chronological reading plan (such as, "Read Chapter 1 during Week 1, Chapter 2 during Week 2," etc.). Instead, my purpose is to equip you with the content that will be most useful to you at each weekly stage.

THE READING PLAN

Session 1:   Preparation and Purpose
Read in *The Daniel Fast*:
- Chapter 1 ("Who Is the Daniel Fast Blogger?")
- Chapter 2 ("Dusting Off an Ancient Spiritual Discipline")
- Frequently Asked Questions
- Review food list, recipes, and meal plans

Session 2:   Fasting and the Body (Fasting Days 1–7)
Read in *The Daniel Fast*:
- Pages 31–42 and 51–54 of Chapter 4 ("The Daniel Fast for Body, Soul, and Spirit")
- Chapter 5 ("Five Steps for a Successful Daniel Fast")
- Continue review of food list, recipes, and meal plans
- Begin the Twenty-One-Day Daniel Fast Devotional

Session 3:   Fasting and the Soul (Fasting Days 8–14)
Read in *The Daniel Fast*:
- Pages 42–46 of Chapter 4 ("The Daniel Fast for Body, Soul, and Spirit")
- Continue the Twenty-One-Day Daniel Fast Devotional

Session 4: Fasting and the Spirit (Fasting Days 15–21)
Read in *The Daniel Fast*:

- Chapter 3 ("Daniel—Determined to Live for God in Enemy Territory")
- Pages 46–51 of Chapter 4 ("The Daniel Fast for Body, Soul, and Spirit")
- Continue and complete the Twenty-One-Day Daniel Fast Devotional

Session 5: Looking Forward after the Daniel Fast
Reread in *The Daniel Fast*:

- Pages 94–95 of Chapter 5 ("Five Steps for a Successful Daniel Fast")

Celebrate and reflect on all you've learned

WHAT YOU'LL FIND EACH WEEK

Within each weekly session, you'll find the following elements (along with a breakdown of how much time to allot for each element if you are meeting as a group; times are based on a 45–60 minute study):

- *The Daniel Fast* reading assignment for that week
- Getting Started: Introductory questions for discussion or reflection (5–10 minutes)
- Core Truths: A summary of the session's theme (5 minutes)
- Setting the Scene: Scripture reading and study questions (10–15 minutes)
- Point to Ponder: A message from *The Daniel Fast* (3 minutes)
- Digging In: Understanding the scriptural application to the fast (10 minutes)

- Discovering and Doing: Practical next steps (10–15 minutes)
- Prayer (2 minutes)
- Tips: Advice for the week (review individually)

If you are fasting as part of a group, that's wonderful! As members of the body of Christ, you will find this to be an amazing spiritual opportunity to encourage, support, and hold each other accountable. Come prepared to discuss what you are feeling, learning, and overcoming through the fasting experience. And, group leaders, don't miss the Leader's Guide at the end of this book, which will help you guide members through the group experience.

Preparation and Purpose

....

READ IN *The Daniel Fast*:

- Chapter 1 ("Who Is the Daniel Fast Blogger?")
- Chapter 2 ("Dusting Off an Ancient Spiritual Discipline")
- Frequently Asked Questions
- Review food list, recipes, and meal plans

GETTING STARTED

- Why have you decided to participate in the Daniel Fast?

- Have you ever fasted before? If so, what challenges and rewards did you experience? If not, what are some anticipations or concerns you have about embarking on the Daniel Fast?

· Fasting is known as a "spiritual discipline." What does that phrase mean to you?

· What questions do you have about the fast? (Don't try to answer them all now, but write down any questions and come back to them at the end of the session.)

CORE TRUTHS: DEFINING YOUR PURPOSE

The better you prepare for the Daniel Fast, the better your experience will be. During this week of planning and preparation before you begin the fast, you will accomplish the following practical steps:

· Decide what you will and will not eat on your Daniel Fast.
· Plan your meals for Week 1.
· Shop for and prepare some of the make-ahead meals for Week 1 of the Daniel Fast.

While much of this week's preparation is focused on food, you'll find the key to a successful fast actually lies much deeper. Here is the most crucial thing you will do this week:

- Ask God to speak to you about your purpose for the Daniel Fast, and invite Him to show you *His* purpose for your life.

When it comes to fasting, a well-established purpose or goal may be the most important thing to get you started on the right track and help you stay there. Your purpose is what will carry you through when your body (or mind) shouts, "Eat!" That's why it's important for your purpose to be personally meaningful. If your goal is not significant enough and compelling to you, it's easy to be tempted to quit or cheat when the going gets tough. But a targeted purpose can carry you through. Here's the simple truth: The more committed you are to your goal or purpose, the more successful you will be on your fast.

Take time during this session to ask God to show you a compelling purpose or goal for your Daniel Fast.

SETTING THE SCENE

Read Daniel 1:5-16 and 10:2-3 and reflect on the experiences of the prophet Daniel upon which we base our fast.

> The king assigned them a daily ration of food and wine from his own kitchens. They were to be trained for three years, and then they would enter the royal service.
> ⁶Daniel, Hananiah, Mishael, and Azariah were four of the young men chosen, all from the tribe of Judah. ⁷The chief of staff renamed them with these Babylonian names:

Daniel was called Belteshazzar.
Hananiah was called Shadrach.
Mishael was called Meshach.
Azariah was called Abednego.

[8]*But Daniel was determined not to defile himself by eating the food and wine given to them by the king. He asked the chief of staff for permission not to eat these unacceptable foods.* [9]*Now God had given the chief of staff both respect and affection for Daniel.* [10]*But he responded, "I am afraid of my lord the king, who has ordered that you eat this food and wine. If you become pale and thin compared to the other youths your age, I am afraid the king will have me beheaded."* [11]*Daniel spoke with the attendant who had been appointed by the chief of staff to look after Daniel, Hananiah, Mishael, and Azariah.* [12]*"Please test us for ten days on a diet of vegetables and water," Daniel said.* [13]*"At the end of the ten days, see how we look compared to the other young men who are eating the king's food. Then make your decision in light of what you see."* [14]*The attendant agreed to Daniel's suggestion and tested them for ten days.*

[15]*At the end of the ten days, Daniel and his three friends looked healthier and better nourished than the young men who had been eating the food assigned by the king.* [16]*So after that, the attendant fed them only vegetables instead of the food and wine provided for the others.*

* * * * * * * * * *

*When this vision came to me, I, Daniel, had been in mourning
for three whole weeks. ³All that time I had eaten no rich food.
No meat or wine crossed my lips, and I used no fragrant lotions
until those three weeks had passed.*

1. What do these passages show us about obedience to God—
   and God's provision for us?

2. How did Daniel's relationship with God inform his decision
   to request a different diet than the one provided by the
   king? How does your own desire for a deeper relationship
   with God inspire you to pursue integrity, boldness, and
   faithfulness?

3. Daniel had a clear, specific purpose in fasting. What does
   this tell us about the importance of being intentional about
   our motives and goals as we fast?

4. What evidence do you see in these passages that God can use our time of fasting to speak and make Himself real to us? What can you do to prepare yourself to *listen* to what God may want to say to you during your fast?

POINT TO PONDER

"Even though you can eat during the Daniel Fast, it is no less effective than a complete fast. The power in fasting has less to do with food than with setting yourself apart for a specific period of time to focus more on the Lord, prayer, and worship. In other words, the power of fasting is found when you consecrate yourself to the Lord and discipline yourself to focus on Him. That's how your spiritual experience is enhanced." (*The Daniel Fast*, Chapter 2)

DIGGING IN

Read Psalm 139, Jeremiah 29:11, and James 1:2-5. As you begin to define your purpose for doing the Daniel Fast, what do these verses reveal about God's investment in your life?

Here are some suggestions you may find helpful in determining the purpose for your fast:

1. Ask God to show you what your purpose should be. After you have prayed, be attentive to how the Holy Spirit might answer you. For example, over the next few days, He may

bring some issues or relationships to mind—or you may find yourself in a situation or a conversation that points you toward a compelling purpose for your fast. One thing is for certain: If you ask God for help, He will be faithful to guide you.

2. What are the top three issues in your life that cause you stress or concern? Ask yourself, *If I could change three things about my life, what would they be?*

3. What five things would you like to accomplish over the next twelve months?

4. What three new habits do you want to form?

5. What fears do you have that you want God to help you conquer?

6. What unforgiveness do you harbor in your heart that you need to deal with?

7. What areas are "out of order" in your life that you need to address?

Now consider your list and select one or two goals as your focus for prayer, study, and action during your Daniel Fast. This will be the purpose for your fast. What goal(s) have you selected?

Write your purpose on a card (or cards) and post it where you will see it regularly throughout the day. You may want to post a card on your bathroom mirror, so it's one of the first things you see each morning, or on your computer monitor, where you can see it as you work. Maybe post a card on the refrigerator or the pantry door. Keeping your purpose firmly in mind will help you stay on track with the Daniel Fast.

DISCOVERING AND DOING

When we're fasting, it's easy to focus on what we're *not* eating or what we *don't* have. The enemy of our souls, Satan, will do everything he can to disrupt and derail our fast. One of his favorite tactics is to combine temptation with subtle suggestions of compromise. Just as he tempted Eve in the Garden of Eden by asking, "Did God really say . . . ?" he may try to tempt you to start questioning the boundaries and principles of the Daniel Fast. That's why it's important to plan your fast and stick to the plan. It's also critical to have your purpose clearly defined and visible throughout the fast.

The more you can prepare in advance—either by planning simple, easy-to-prepare meals or cooking ahead and freezing meals—the easier the twenty-one days of the fast will be. Don't become so concerned with meal plans and recipes that they become the primary focus of your planning and preparation. Remember, the key to a successful fast is getting your mind *off* the food and *onto* God. By establishing your food list and planning your meals in advance, you can eliminate a lot of the day-to-day decisions you'll have to make during the fast. The more you have planned in advance, the more productive the days of the fast will be.

Too much emphasis on recipes and meal plans can make the whole process seem daunting, but don't forget that the Daniel Fast lasts for only *three weeks*. If you simplify your menu by focusing on easy-to-prepare fruits, vegetables, and whole grains, the planning process shouldn't be difficult. And if you have identified and committed to your purpose, you will find yourself relying on God's will for you to get through the "valley" moments of fasting and enjoy the "peaks" of its many rewards.

1. What plans will you make this week for choosing and eating the right foods? (See *The Daniel Fast* for recipes and menus.)

2. What foods will you eat? Which ones will you avoid? Which recipes sound like ones you might want to try first?

3. What practical steps do you need to take this week (meal planning, grocery shopping, cooking ahead of time) to make sure you are well prepared to begin on day 1 of the fast?

4. One of the benefits of fasting is that it takes us out of our normal routines and creates an opportunity for us to reflect on our relationship with God and better connect with Him. But it won't just happen. We need to *decide*. How will you pray, meditate, and study during your fast?

5. Your plan should include establishing a specific time and place to have a one-on-one interaction with God, where interruptions and distractions are minimized. What is your time and place for Bible study and prayer?

6. It's not helpful to focus your attention on how you're feeling during a fast. But you *will* be feeling things (especially if you're new to fasting). Prepare for this by anticipating where you might be weak or vulnerable—and have a plan in place

for how you're going to deal with it. For example, you may want to ask a friend to encourage you to "stay the course" if you are tempted to quit or cheat. Who might that person be? Will you reach out and ask him or her to be available to you over the course of your fast? In addition to being a "phone call away," your accountability partner should be someone who will pray for you as you fast.

7. What will you do during the twenty-one days of the fast to supplement your healthy eating with stretching and exercise? Write a specific plan.

8. What will you do during the twenty-one days of the fast to reduce your stress and get plenty of rest? Write a specific plan.

PRAYER

Father, as we prepare our bodies and minds for a time of focusing more deeply on You, we pray that You will clear the path for us. Help us to continually choose You as we make our daily decisions about what to eat and how to spend our time and energy. Equip us this week with the gift of preparation as we think ahead to the next twenty-one days and consider them a special and holy time set apart. And bless us with a strong sense of Your purpose—both for the goal that will carry us through the fast, and the abiding knowledge of Your will for our lives. Amen.

TIPS

- Starting today, begin tapering off your consumption of caffeine, sugar, and other foods not on the Daniel Fast. For example, you may want to progressively reduce the amount of coffee you drink each day or switch to half-caff or decaf.
- Each day, be sure to drink at least half a gallon (sixty-four ounces) of pure, filtered water.
- Get plenty of rest and a moderate amount of exercise.
- You may find it helpful to remove items from your pantry that you won't be using during the Daniel Fast and put them in a secure place out of the way. I call this "locking up our weaknesses." When trying to change or control the way we eat, the first line of defense is always availability. It's often easier to avoid temptation altogether than to rely on our ability to resist it. Also, planning your meals and knowing what you will eat plays a significant role in complying with the fast.
- To receive free resources, including the Daniel Fast Food List and Guidelines, the Daniel Fast Weekly Meal Planning Worksheet, and other helpful tools, go to www.daniel-fast.com. Enter your name and e-mail address in the form provided, and I'll send you the information right away.

Fasting and the Body

(Fasting Days 1–7)

....

READ IN *The Daniel Fast*:

- Pages 31–42 and 51–54 of Chapter 4 ("The Daniel Fast for Body, Soul, and Spirit")
- Chapter 5 ("Five Steps for a Successful Daniel Fast")
- Continue review of food list, recipes, and meal plans
- Begin the Twenty-One-Day Daniel Fast Devotional

GETTING STARTED

- How would you define the differences between the Daniel Fast and a simple diet or weight-loss plan?

- What are some reasons we should take care of our bodies? How and why do you think our bodies are important to God?

- How do you anticipate your body might react to your dietary changes during Week 1 of the Daniel Fast? How might it be reacting by Week 3?

- As you begin the fast, is there a part of it you are particularly excited about? Anxious about?

CORE TRUTHS: YOUR BODY

During the twenty-one days of the Daniel Fast, you will take time for Bible study, reflection, and prayer. I also encourage you to use the Twenty-One-Day Daniel Fast Devotional (found in *The Daniel Fast*) as an anchor point for your daily quiet time. Remember, all of these tools and resources are meant to be *interactive*—between you and God. Allow Him to speak to you, and be sure to listen for His encouragement, insight, and guidance.

The Daniel Fast touches on the whole person—body, soul, and spirit. This week we'll be focusing on the body, and you will

- think about why your body has value;
- develop a plan for how you can treat your body with greater respect; and
- be prepared to notice (and write down) how God helps you overcome your physical desires and cravings.

We all know that our culture can be obsessed with the external. From magazines to movies to weight-loss plans, our focus is glued to what our eyes can see. Far too often, we gauge someone's worth (or our own) by things like waistline, attractiveness, or clothing. Yet the Bible tells us we are so much more than this! Our bodies are immensely valuable—but not because of their appearance. Instead, they have value because they are dwelling places of God.

We're used to allowing our physical needs to dictate almost everything we do. When we're tired, we sleep—or consume caffeine to help us stay awake. When we're hungry, bored, or upset, we eat. When we have a craving for a treat, we indulge our taste buds. Yet the process of fasting brings the body back to its rightful place: under the control of the spirit. When we're fasting, we are willing to deny ourselves because that encourages us to turn to God.

SETTING THE SCENE

Read Daniel 3:1-30. In this passage, Daniel's three friends, Shadrach, Meshach, and Abednego, take center stage. As you read, consider the source of their remarkable courage.

King Nebuchadnezzar made a gold statue ninety feet tall and nine feet wide and set it up on the plain of Dura in the province of Babylon. ²Then he sent messages to the high officers, officials, governors, advisers, treasurers, judges, magistrates, and all the provincial officials to come to the dedication of the statue he had set up. ³So all these officials came and stood before the statue King Nebuchadnezzar had set up.

⁴Then a herald shouted out, "People of all races and nations and languages, listen to the king's command! ⁵When you hear the sound of the horn, flute, zither, lyre, harp, pipes, and other musical instruments, bow to the ground to worship King Nebuchadnezzar's gold statue. ⁶Anyone who refuses to obey will immediately be thrown into a blazing furnace."

⁷So at the sound of the musical instruments, all the people, whatever their race or nation or language, bowed to the ground and worshiped the gold statue that King Nebuchadnezzar had set up.

⁸But some of the astrologers went to the king and informed on the Jews. ⁹They said to King Nebuchadnezzar, "Long live the king! ¹⁰You issued a decree requiring all the people to bow down and worship the gold statue when they hear the sound of the horn, flute, zither, lyre, harp, pipes, and other musical instruments. ¹¹That decree also states that those who refuse to obey must be thrown into a blazing furnace. ¹²But there are some Jews—Shadrach, Meshach, and Abednego—whom you have put in charge of the province of Babylon. They pay no attention to you, Your Majesty. They refuse to serve your gods and do not worship the gold statue you have set up."

¹³Then Nebuchadnezzar flew into a rage and ordered that Shadrach, Meshach, and Abednego be brought before him. When they were brought in, ¹⁴Nebuchadnezzar said to them, "Is it true, Shadrach, Meshach, and Abednego, that you refuse to serve my gods or to worship the gold statue I have set up? [15]*I will give you one more chance to bow down and worship the statue I have made when you hear the sound of the musical instruments. But if you refuse, you will be thrown immediately into the blazing furnace. And then what god will be able to rescue you from my power?"*

[16]*Shadrach, Meshach, and Abednego replied, "O Nebuchadnezzar, we do not need to defend ourselves before you. [17]If we are thrown into the blazing furnace, the God whom we serve is able to save us. He will rescue us from your power, Your Majesty. [18]But even if he doesn't, we want to make it clear to you, Your Majesty, that we will never serve your gods or worship the gold statue you have set up."*

[19]*Nebuchadnezzar was so furious with Shadrach, Meshach, and Abednego that his face became distorted with rage. He commanded that the furnace be heated seven times hotter than usual. [20]Then he ordered some of the strongest men of his army to bind Shadrach, Meshach, and Abednego and throw them into the blazing furnace. [21]So they tied them up and threw them into the furnace, fully dressed in their pants, turbans, robes, and other garments. [22]And because the king, in his anger, had demanded such a hot fire in the furnace, the flames killed the soldiers as they threw the three men in. [23]So Shadrach, Meshach, and Abednego, securely tied, fell into the roaring flames.*

[24]*But suddenly, Nebuchadnezzar jumped up in amazement and exclaimed to his advisers, "Didn't we tie up three men and throw them into the furnace?"*

"Yes, Your Majesty, we certainly did," they replied.

²⁵ *"Look!" Nebuchadnezzar shouted. "I see four men, unbound, walking around in the fire unharmed! And the fourth looks like a god!"*

²⁶ *Then Nebuchadnezzar came as close as he could to the door of the flaming furnace and shouted: "Shadrach, Meshach, and Abednego, servants of the Most High God, come out! Come here!"*

So Shadrach, Meshach, and Abednego stepped out of the fire. ²⁷ Then the high officers, officials, governors, and advisers crowded around them and saw that the fire had not touched them. Not a hair on their heads was singed, and their clothing was not scorched. They didn't even smell of smoke!

²⁸ *Then Nebuchadnezzar said, "Praise to the God of Shadrach, Meshach, and Abednego! He sent his angel to rescue his servants who trusted in him. They defied the king's command and were willing to die rather than serve or worship any god except their own God. ²⁹ Therefore, I make this decree: If any people, whatever their race or nation or language, speak a word against the God of Shadrach, Meshach, and Abednego, they will be torn limb from limb, and their houses will be turned into heaps of rubble. There is no other god who can rescue like this!"*

³⁰ *Then the king promoted Shadrach, Meshach, and Abednego to even higher positions in the province of Babylon.*

1. When faced with a choice that could lead to devastating consequences, Shadrach, Meshach, and Abednego didn't hesitate to do the right thing. What do you think was the

source of their courage? What training and habits might have prepared them for this moment?

2. It's clear from both this passage and Daniel 1, which we read during Week 1, that Shadrach, Meshach, and Abednego had a defined life purpose: to serve God. How do you think this purpose helped them when they faced this difficult test?

3. It's human nature to put a huge priority on preserving our bodies. What enabled the three young men to look beyond their physical safety? What are some situations where you need to look beyond your physical circumstances to the deeper reality of spiritual things?

4. Reflect on the faith behind the statement from the three young men found in verses 16-18. What does it mean to step out in faith even without a guarantee that God will save you? In what areas of your life are you being challenged to act on faith?

5. How can the courage and steadfastness of these young men encourage you this week in your fast?

POINT TO PONDER

"Christ calls us to walk according to the Spirit and not the flesh. We are to crucify our flesh—all those worldly thoughts and emotions—and allow the Holy Spirit to guide us and direct us.

"That's the way Daniel and his companions lived their lives. They were sold out to God, and they filled their minds, hearts, and words with Him and His ways. When Nebuchadnezzar threatened to throw Shadrach, Meshach, and Abednego into the fiery furnace, their faith was so strong they didn't even flinch." (*The Daniel Fast*, Chapter 4)

DIGGING IN

Shadrach, Meshach, and Abednego are powerful models for a deeply rooted faith. When faced with the threat of being thrown into the fiery furnace, they held strong to their faith in the God who cared for them and whom they loved. They knew God. They trusted Him. And their faith was so firmly established that nothing could sway them. This unwavering faith didn't come quickly. Every day each young man opened his heart to God, submitted himself to Him, and lived according to His ways. This "lifestyle" spawned security, freedom, and confidence and became their identity.

When we submit and bring our bodies under the control of our spirits, we experience freedom. We no longer need to be obsessed with our appearance, and we don't have to live in fear of the physical changes or illnesses we might experience on earth. We are free to take exceptional care of our bodies for the best possible reason: because they are God's dwelling place! Caring for our bodies means being aware of the food we eat, the amount of rest and exercise we get, and even the way we think about our physical selves. We can honor God by treating our bodies with respect and by taking care of them so that we have more energy and focus for God's work. Yet we can also know—and be filled with gratitude—that our identity encompasses more than just what we can see.

DISCOVERING AND DOING

As you dive into Week 1 of the fast, your body will let you know that it misses its regular food. As you deal with temptations to break the fast, keep reminding yourself of the body's proper place: under the control of the spirit. Feel the freedom that comes from not letting your body be in charge. When you experience hunger or cravings, thank God for your body and ask Him to help you view it with the right perspective.

1. In the last lesson, we noted that your plan should include establishing a time and a quiet place to have one-on-one fellowship with God. How has that been working so far? If you have had interruptions and distractions, what can you do to improve the atmosphere and setting to better help you concentrate?

2. On page 34 of *The Daniel Fast*, we read this about Shadrach, Meshach, and Abednego: "This wasn't a faith built from Sunday morning church attendance and prayers over their meals. This was a deeply rooted faith in God they had developed by filling their souls with God's Word and truth on a daily basis." How might the fast be an opportunity for you to go deeper in your Bible study, to *feast* on God's Word?

3. In the last lesson, you recorded your goals for the fast. If you meet those goals, how do you hope and pray that will affect your family? Your church? Your workplace? Your neighborhood and community?

4. Reflect on your physical experience so far. What adjustments might you need to make to your food choices or preparation to make the experience easier for you?

5. Fasting brings our bodily desires to the forefront. What are you discovering about your body? What do you often think of as *needs* that are actually *wants*?

6. Read 1 Corinthians 6:19-20. What does it mean for your body to be a "temple of the Holy Spirit"? How can you change the ways you treat your body—whether through what you eat or your habits of exercise, rest, and use of time—to better respect its purpose?

PRAYER

Father, in this first week of the fast, we want to set our minds on You. We pray that our physical discomforts or cravings will not distract us from our intended purpose, but instead will turn us to You. In these weeks we want to be consecrated—set apart—for You and Your purposes. May we find joy in the constant reminders that we are Yours and that our bodies are Your temple. Encourage us to be steadfast in our purpose, keeping in mind our goal of having a closer relationship with You. We pray for the self-discipline to persevere when things are difficult, seeking Your will most of all. Amen.

TIPS

- Develop a plan to help you deal with temptations. Consider writing down Scripture verses and putting them in key places, where they will remind you to think past the temporary urges of your body and instead focus on its ultimate purpose. Try 1 Corinthians 6:19 or Romans 12:1.
- Fatigue, headaches, cramps, and joint pain are common side effects of detoxing from caffeine and sugar. If you are

experiencing these symptoms, try increasing your water intake. You'll want to drink at least sixty-four ounces of water each day. To be even more precise, a good rule of thumb is to divide your body weight by two and drink that number of ounces each day (e.g., a 160-pound person would drink eighty ounces of water daily).

- Continue to get plenty of rest and moderate exercise.
- There are many adjustments to make in the first week of the fast, and you may find yourself overly focused on the details of what you can and cannot eat. If food is consuming your thoughts and distracting you from the spiritual purpose of the fast, try doing more meal planning and preparing food ahead of time. That will allow your days to go more smoothly and give you more time to devote to prayer.
- If you have questions about foods you can or cannot eat, visit the blog or FAQ page at www.daniel-fast.com.
- Remember, set yourself up for success. Plan a quiet time of prayer and Bible study that encourages, motivates, and feeds your soul. Use this time of extended prayer and fasting to develop life-giving habits that will help you beyond the twenty-one days of the Daniel Fast.

Fasting and the Soul

(Fasting Days 8–14)

....

READ IN *The Daniel Fast*:

- Pages 42–46 of Chapter 4 ("The Daniel Fast for Body, Soul, and Spirit")
- Continue the Twenty-One-Day Daniel Fast Devotional

GETTING STARTED

- Reflect on Week 1 of the fast. What were the biggest challenges, physically and spiritually? What were the most significant rewards? What surprised you?

- Review the purpose you established for the fast. Have you gained insights as you have prayed and studied God's Word? Have you experienced lessons while fasting that you didn't expect?

- Fasting can bring to light some places where our souls, or flesh, govern areas of our lives. How have you found that to be true this week?

CORE TRUTHS: YOUR SOUL

As you move into the second week of the Daniel Fast, you may notice the challenges becoming less strictly physical and more emotional and spiritual. In this session, we focus on the soul, or flesh—the part of our being that houses our conscience, emotions, personality, intellect, and will. This week you will

- think about what it means to be transformed by God;
- view moments of temptation as opportunities for growth; and
- consider in what areas you want your soul to submit more fully to God.

Our constant challenge as humans and believers in Christ is to let His Spirit—not our own worldly trained flesh—be in control of our lives. Fasting can make us aware of this struggle in a dramatic way. When we choose to fast (to limit certain foods for a spiritual purpose), we suddenly come face-to-face with our own weaknesses. Yet those very moments when we are most tempted to cheat or quit altogether are the moments that point the way to transformation. In Romans 12:2, Paul encourages us to be transformed by renewing our minds. When we change our attitudes and conform to God's Word—rather than to the world around us or to our temporary circumstances—we will become more and more mature in Christ.

How do we renew our minds? By saturating them with God's Word so we can gain revelation from His truth. By devoting ourselves to prayer and developing a deeper intimacy with our Father. By letting God change our perspective little by little, until some of the things we once thought were so important fade away in the light of what God wants to accomplish in our lives.

SETTING THE SCENE

Daniel spent decades of his life in an alien society that opposed much of what he stood for. Yet, although he became a powerful adviser to the king, he did not conform to the surrounding culture. Through his disciplines of prayer and time in Scripture, he was continually being transformed into the person God had called him to be. Read again Daniel 6, the familiar story about how Daniel reacted with faith at a point of crisis.

> *Darius the Mede decided to divide the kingdom into 120 provinces, and he appointed a high officer to rule over each province. [2] The king also chose Daniel and two others as administrators to supervise the high officers and protect the king's interests. [3] Daniel soon proved himself more capable*

than all the other administrators and high officers. Because
of Daniel's great ability, the king made plans to place him
over the entire empire.

⁴Then the other administrators and high officers began
searching for some fault in the way Daniel was handling
government affairs, but they couldn't find anything to criticize
or condemn. He was faithful, always responsible, and completely
trustworthy. ⁵So they concluded, "Our only chance of finding
grounds for accusing Daniel will be in connection with the rules
of his religion."

⁶So the administrators and high officers went to the king and
said, "Long live King Darius! ⁷We are all in agreement—we
administrators, officials, high officers, advisers, and governors—
that the king should make a law that will be strictly enforced.
Give orders that for the next thirty days any person who prays to
anyone, divine or human—except to you, Your Majesty—will
be thrown into the den of lions. ⁸And now, Your Majesty, issue
and sign this law so it cannot be changed, an official law of the
Medes and Persians that cannot be revoked." ⁹So King Darius
signed the law.

¹⁰But when Daniel learned that the law had been signed,
he went home and knelt down as usual in his upstairs room,
with its windows open toward Jerusalem. He prayed three times
a day, just as he had always done, giving thanks to his God.
¹¹Then the officials went together to Daniel's house and found
him praying and asking for God's help. ¹²So they went straight
to the king and reminded him about his law. "Did you not
sign a law that for the next thirty days any person who prays

to anyone, divine or human—except to you, Your Majesty—will be thrown into the den of lions?"

"Yes," the king replied, "that decision stands; it is an official law of the Medes and Persians that cannot be revoked."

¹³*Then they told the king, "That man Daniel, one of the captives from Judah, is ignoring you and your law. He still prays to his God three times a day."*

¹⁴*Hearing this, the king was deeply troubled, and he tried to think of a way to save Daniel. He spent the rest of the day looking for a way to get Daniel out of this predicament.*

¹⁵*In the evening the men went together to the king and said, "Your Majesty, you know that according to the law of the Medes and the Persians, no law that the king signs can be changed."*

¹⁶*So at last the king gave orders for Daniel to be arrested and thrown into the den of lions. The king said to him, "May your God, whom you serve so faithfully, rescue you."*

¹⁷*A stone was brought and placed over the mouth of the den. The king sealed the stone with his own royal seal and the seals of his nobles, so that no one could rescue Daniel.* ¹⁸*Then the king returned to his palace and spent the night fasting. He refused his usual entertainment and couldn't sleep at all that night.*

¹⁹*Very early the next morning, the king got up and hurried out to the lions' den.* ²⁰*When he got there, he called out in anguish, "Daniel, servant of the living God! Was your God, whom you serve so faithfully, able to rescue you from the lions?"*

²¹*Daniel answered, "Long live the king!* ²²*My God sent his angel to shut the lions' mouths so that they would not hurt me, for I have been found innocent in his sight. And I have not wronged you, Your Majesty."*

²³ *The king was overjoyed and ordered that Daniel be lifted from the den. Not a scratch was found on him, for he had trusted in his God.*

²⁴ *Then the king gave orders to arrest the men who had maliciously accused Daniel. He had them thrown into the lions' den, along with their wives and children. The lions leaped on them and tore them apart before they even hit the floor of the den.*

²⁵ *Then King Darius sent this message to the people of every race and nation and language throughout the world:*

"Peace and prosperity to you!
²⁶ *"I decree that everyone throughout my kingdom should tremble with fear before the God of Daniel.*

For he is the living God,
  and he will endure forever.
His kingdom will never be destroyed,
  and his rule will never end.
²⁷ *He rescues and saves his people;*
  he performs miraculous signs and wonders
  in the heavens and on earth.
He has rescued Daniel
  from the power of the lions."

²⁸ *So Daniel prospered during the reign of Darius and the reign of Cyrus the Persian.*

1. What does Daniel's response to the king's new law tell us about him? What does it tell us about qualities that God finds pleasing in us? How does the Daniel Fast provide the opportunity to call out and strengthen such qualities?

2. Daniel was not spared from entering the lions' den, but he was kept safe in a seemingly impossible situation. What does Daniel's experience show us about the way God meets us in the midst of our trials? How might this apply to our daily experiences on the Daniel Fast?

3. What was the secret of Daniel's strong faith and his close relationship with God (verses 10-11)? In what specific ways do we see that Daniel's actions were informed by God's Word, not by his own flesh?

4. Daniel's faith and God's response so impressed King Darius that he made a remarkable proclamation about Daniel's God (verses 25-27). How might your example of stalwart faith in the face of challenges influence those around you?

5. The key to Daniel's success was his faithfulness in prayer. What pressures, interests, and activities tend to interfere with your prayer life? What can you do to spend consistent, quality time in prayer?

POINT TO PONDER

"God didn't keep Daniel from ever entering the lions' den, just like He didn't keep Daniel's companions from being thrown into the fiery furnace (see Daniel 3). But God met them in the midst of their calamities and delivered them." (*The Daniel Fast*, Chapter 3)

DIGGING IN

As a man who had served God faithfully for decades, Daniel must have been well aware of the human tendency to let our souls—the flesh—take over. He lived and worked among royal advisers (or "wise men") who elevated human reason above all else, and Daniel was the wisest of them all. He could have trusted in his own intellect, but instead, through consistent prayer and time in Scripture, he let his mind be renewed by God. Then, when a huge challenge came his way, he was prepared to step out in faith.

Scripture makes it clear that trials are opportunities for growth. Romans 5:3-5 says, "We can rejoice, too, when we run into problems and trials, for we know that they help us develop endurance. And endurance develops strength of character, and character strengthens our confident hope of salvation. And this hope will not lead to disappointment. For we know how dearly God loves us, because he has given us the Holy Spirit to fill our hearts with his love."

When we're fasting, every craving or temptation is an opportunity to develop perseverance and self-discipline. How empowering to approach problems that way! We are not at the mercy of our emotions, we're not limited by our human perspective, and we're not trapped by our desires. We do not have to let our flesh rule us! We can look right at that piece of chocolate we're tempted to eat and say, "Thank You, Lord, for teaching me perseverance right now." We can use those temptations as reminders to pray and immerse ourselves in Scripture. We can train ourselves to look beyond what we want in this moment and look ahead to what we want long-term: a character that is transformed by God.

- How can viewing struggles as opportunities for growth help change your attitude toward problems?

- Think of a few scenarios where you are tempted. What do you hope to gain short-term? What long-term benefits to your character might you experience if you resisted?

DISCOVERING AND DOING

When we're fasting, the pull of the flesh is very evident. Our human nature will try to take control of what we're doing. Yet we're not helpless. Like Daniel, we can submit our whole being to God and pursue transformation through the disciplines of prayer and Scripture reading.

1. Review your plan for spending time with God in Bible study and prayer. How has that worked so far? Remember that fasting is not just about limiting food—it's about entering a focused time of spiritual discovery and growth. Renew your commitment to make your fast a time of spiritual transformation. Take time every day to come to the Lord, asking Him to renew your mind. Bask in the Scriptures and ask God to help them penetrate your heart and change your thinking.

2. Think about the parts of your life where you want to submit more fully to God. Ask Him to reveal the areas in which you need to be transformed. These might be specific attitudes or thought patterns about your family, your work, your purpose, your finances, or how you use your time.

3. The soul is where our feelings are located. As you go through this week, pay attention to the effects your emotions have on you, both positive and negative. What triggers your strongest feelings? How can you regain mastery over your emotions?

4. When are you most tempted to break your fast? Prepare for these moments by remembering that they can be opportunities to develop your character. It may help you to write out Romans 5:3-5 and put it in your kitchen or somewhere else where you may be tempted. Read it out loud when you are dealing with a craving or have lost your sense of purpose for the fast.

You'll want to develop and create a daily time of focused praise, prayer, study, and reflection. In Romans 1:21, we see how Paul describes the behavior of those who don't have a relationship with God: "Yes, they knew God, but they wouldn't worship him as God or even give him thanks. And they began to think up foolish ideas of what God was like. As a result, their minds became dark and confused."

Clearly, we want to do the opposite. I like to use these four simple steps to keep my mind and heart fixed on God and His goodness:

- **Glorify God** by acknowledging His greatness, which is evident in my surroundings and encounters.
- **Be thankful** to the Lord for all He is doing in my life, in the lives of those I love, and in my circumstances.
- **Know God** by studying His Word, opening my heart to Him, and praying with a submitted and receptive mind.
- **Renew my mind** to the ways of God so that I can learn, grow, and follow His ways.

Make sure to allow time to *listen* to God as He shares His truth with you. After you pray, stop and quiet your heart. Be sensitive to what the Holy Spirit impresses on you.

PRAYER

Father, this week we are so aware of how often our flesh rules us. It affects the way we think, what we feel, what we eat, and how we respond to others. But we don't want our lives to be ruled by our self-centered wants. We want them to reflect our love for You! Please help us this week to begin to understand how You are transforming us into Your image and how we can submit to that process. Give us the grace to approach problems with hope, knowing that they are opportunities for us to grow and change. Thank You that You are faithful and that You are working in our lives. May we be blessed this week through the Daniel Fast. Amen.

TIPS

- Keep reviewing your goals and your purpose for the fast each day. This will give you strength to persevere through the remaining days.
- Some people are concerned because they don't feel deprived on the Daniel Fast. That's a wonderful problem, because it means you're retraining your taste buds to enjoy healthy foods. Remember, you don't have to suffer for the fast to be effective. The important thing is to discipline yourself to eat only certain foods and to make sure you're doing it for a spiritual purpose.
- If you're on a budget, remember that meal planning is the key to keeping food costs down. Also, because you're not buying

processed food, you'll have more money freed up to purchase fresh produce.

- If you find yourself overly focused on food because you're hungry or experiencing cravings, increase your time in the Word to maintain your spiritual focus.
- If you slip up and accidentally eat something you're not supposed to, see this as a mistake or a temporary setback. Make a note of it so you can avoid it next time, and get yourself back on track.
- Don't be surprised if the flesh rebels against your attempts to bring it under the control of the spirit. Jesus said, "The spirit is willing, but the body is weak!" (Matthew 26:41). If you've purposely cheated on the fast, don't give up. Consider why you chose to depart from the fasting guidelines. Confess it to God, forgive yourself, and then determine to make a new start and continue on with the fast as planned.

Fasting and the Spirit

(Fasting Days 15–21)

READ IN *The Daniel Fast*:

- Chapter 3 ("Daniel—Determined to Live for God in Enemy Territory")
- Pages 46–51 of Chapter 4 ("The Daniel Fast for Body, Soul, and Spirit")
- Continue and complete the Twenty-One-Day Daniel Fast Devotional

GETTING STARTED

- Reflect on Week 2 of the fast. What were the biggest challenges and rewards? What worked well for you this week, and where did you struggle?

- How are you doing on the goals you set for the fast? What could you do differently this week to help you reach them more effectively?

- How do you typically respond when you have a hunger twinge or a craving? How do you think this fits in with your overall spiritual life?

- What does it mean to walk in the Spirit? Describe a time in your life when you felt like you were doing this.

- In what areas do you most struggle with letting the Holy Spirit take control of your life?

CORE TRUTHS: YOUR SPIRIT

As you are experiencing, the Daniel Fast affects the whole person: body, soul, and spirit. Your body needs to be respected as a temple of the Holy Spirit. Your soul, or flesh, needs to be put in the right position so that it does not run your life. And your spirit needs to be strengthened day by day so you live the way God intended you to. But how do you strengthen your spirit—what I call the "God-centered essence where Christ abides"? And how do you know when you have made progress? That's what we'll look at this week. You will

- think about what it means to walk by the Spirit;
- strengthen your spirit through choosing to focus on God; and
- remember that it's not all up to you; the Holy Spirit is working.

The Holy Spirit is the key. When Jesus left this earth, He told His disciples that a Helper would come to them—the Holy Spirit, the Spirit of truth. And as believers in Christ whose spirits have been born again, we have access to that Spirit! He is living within us, and He will guide us, if we are willing. Every day we have a choice: Will we live according to the flesh and gratify our own desires, or will we live according to the Spirit? Will we be focused on ourselves, or will we be focused on Christ?

As we finish this last week of the Daniel Fast, we have the opportunity to make these choices. Think of these last days as a training ground, making our spirits stronger with each choice to let the Holy Spirit be in control. As we deny ourselves certain foods for a spiritual purpose, we will begin to see how exciting our lives can be when our flesh steps out of the way. When we turn to God in prayer at each temptation, He will become even more real to us. As we submit ourselves to the Spirit, we will grow ever stronger in the knowledge of Christ.

SETTING THE SCENE

Read Daniel 2:1-23.

One night during the second year of his reign, Nebuchadnezzar had such disturbing dreams that he couldn't sleep. ² *He called in his magicians, enchanters, sorcerers, and astrologers, and he demanded that they tell him what he had dreamed. As they stood before the king,* ³ *he said, "I have had a dream that deeply troubles me, and I must know what it means."*

⁴ *Then the astrologers answered the king in Aramaic, "Long live the king! Tell us the dream, and we will tell you what it means."*

⁵ *But the king said to the astrologers, "I am serious about this. If you don't tell me what my dream was and what it means, you will be torn limb from limb, and your houses will be turned into heaps of rubble!* ⁶ *But if you tell me what I dreamed and what the dream means, I will give you many wonderful gifts and honors. Just tell me the dream and what it means!"*

⁷ *They said again, "Please, Your Majesty. Tell us the dream, and we will tell you what it means."*

⁸ *The king replied, "I know what you are doing! You're stalling for time because you know I am serious when I say,* ⁹ *'If you don't tell me the dream, you are doomed.' So you have conspired to tell me lies, hoping I will change my mind. But tell me the dream, and then I'll know that you can tell me what it means."*

¹⁰ *The astrologers replied to the king, "No one on earth can tell the king his dream! And no king, however great*

and powerful, has ever asked such a thing of any magician, enchanter, or astrologer! ¹¹*The king's demand is impossible. No one except the gods can tell you your dream, and they do not live here among people."*

¹²*The king was furious when he heard this, and he ordered that all the wise men of Babylon be executed.* ¹³*And because of the king's decree, men were sent to find and kill Daniel and his friends.*

¹⁴*When Arioch, the commander of the king's guard, came to kill them, Daniel handled the situation with wisdom and discretion.* ¹⁵*He asked Arioch, "Why has the king issued such a harsh decree?" So Arioch told him all that had happened.* ¹⁶*Daniel went at once to see the king and requested more time to tell the king what the dream meant.*

¹⁷*Then Daniel went home and told his friends Hananiah, Mishael, and Azariah what had happened.* ¹⁸*He urged them to ask the God of heaven to show them his mercy by telling them the secret, so they would not be executed along with the other wise men of Babylon.* ¹⁹*That night the secret was revealed to Daniel in a vision. Then Daniel praised the God of heaven.* ²⁰*He said,*

"Praise the name of God forever and ever,
for he has all wisdom and power.
²¹*He controls the course of world events;*
he removes kings and sets up other kings.
He gives wisdom to the wise
and knowledge to the scholars.

> ²²*He reveals deep and mysterious things*
>   *and knows what lies hidden in darkness,*
>   *though he is surrounded by light.*
> ²³*I thank and praise you, God of my ancestors,*
>   *for you have given me wisdom and strength.*
>   *You have told me what we asked of you*
>   *and revealed to us what the king demanded."*

1. Daniel and all the wise men were confronted with a demand that, in human terms, seemed impossible: to tell the king his dream and then interpret it. Contrast the other wise men's response with Daniel's. Why were they so different?

2. In what specific ways does Daniel's response show his dependence on God's power?

3. Reread Daniel's prayer of praise (verses 20-23). What does it tell us about God's character? What does it reveal about Daniel?

4. How does Daniel's prayer give us perspective on our place in God's plan?

5. Later, in verse 47, after Daniel reveals the dream and its interpretation to Nebuchadnezzar, the king responds with amazement—not at Daniel, but at God's power: "Truly, your God is the greatest of gods, the Lord over kings, a revealer of mysteries, for you have been able to reveal this secret." How can our choice to walk in the Spirit point others not to us but to the God we serve?

POINT TO PONDER

"[We] have a lot in common with Daniel and the other Hebrew men. As believers, we are also in enemy territory, facing the pressures of this world. And just like Daniel, we can choose to live according to God's ways—not just when it's convenient and not in a casual way. If we want what Daniel had, we must be willing to do what Daniel did. . . .

"Daniel's faith brought him through. His life lived for God is why [we] are even giving him attention today! And his life of unwavering faith is why he serves as a worthy example for us as we enter into a powerful period of prayer and fasting unto the Lord." (*The Daniel Fast*, Chapter 3)

DIGGING IN

When Daniel discovered that his life was in danger again, he didn't panic. He didn't respond in any of the ways his flesh would have encouraged, such as bemoaning his circumstances or demanding that

God explain *why* he was experiencing such troubles. He simply prayed, and he recruited his friends to pray too. They sought God's mercy, and when He responded, Daniel praised Him—not just for saving Daniel and his friends from death, but for who He was. Daniel knew that no matter what his circumstances, God was sovereign and faithful.

When we're living in the Spirit, we're able to live in the way God intended. We are in communion with God, fulfilling His purpose for our lives and being led by Him.

- Take a moment to think about God's great love for you. About His design for your life. And about how very much He values you. What can you do to step into the fullness of who you are as a precious child of God?

- Ask God to reveal the areas where you most need to let His character change the way you think and live. Write down those areas and think about how you can surrender them to God.

- One way to train yourself to think more deeply about God is to meditate on Scripture passages that reveal His attributes—such as His love, faithfulness, justice, holiness, and righteousness. Sometime this week, consider using a concordance or a keyword search to find applicable passages, and then journal about them.

Galatians 2:20 says, "My old self has been crucified with Christ. It is no longer I who live, but Christ lives in me. So I live in this earthly body by trusting in the Son of God, who loved me and gave himself for me." When we walk in the Spirit, we remember that our old self is gone. It no longer controls us! Now we live by faith, in Christ. And as we make that choice each day—or each moment, each decision of each day—we'll find our spirits growing stronger.

DISCOVERING AND DOING

Walking in the Spirit is a daily choice. Yet it is not merely about willpower. Consider Galatians 5:22-25:

> *The Holy Spirit produces this kind of fruit in our lives: love, joy, peace, patience, kindness, goodness, faithfulness, gentleness, and self-control. There is no law against these things!*
>
> *Those who belong to Christ Jesus have nailed the passions and desires of their sinful nature to his cross and crucified them there. Since we are living by the Spirit, let us follow the Spirit's leading in every part of our lives.*

The "fruit" listed in this passage is called "of the Spirit" because it is produced *by* Him! Our job is not to try harder and harder to do the right things or have the right attitudes. No, our job is to choose to submit ourselves to the Spirit and allow Him to do His work in us.

As you work through these last seven days of the fast, I encourage you to keep this thought at the forefront of your mind: *The Holy Spirit is working in you!* Pray that you will be wholly available to Him and open to His work. Remember that doing this fast—or any other act of service to God—cannot make Him love you any more. You are His child! You are His in Christ. It is because He loves you that He wants to make you more and more like Christ—more and more who you were created to be.

1. When are you tempted to think that having better willpower is the key to living in the Spirit? Does this mind-set make you feel encouraged or discouraged? How can you change your focus this week from relying on willpower alone to allowing the Holy Spirit to work?

2. Think back on the past weeks of the fast. What changes have you seen in yourself? Can you point to places where you know the Holy Spirit was working? Use these experiences to help you remember that He is faithful, even when we are not.

3. What can you do this last week of the fast to keep your attention focused on God and His character rather than on yourself?

Consider meditating on some of the following verses, which will remind you of your identity in Christ and His faithful love for you:

- "I am certain that God, who began the good work within you, will continue his work until it is finally finished on the day when Christ Jesus returns." (Philippians 1:6)
- "I am convinced that nothing can ever separate us from God's love. Neither death nor life, neither angels nor demons, neither our fears for today nor our worries about tomorrow— not even the powers of hell can separate us from God's love. No power in the sky above or in the earth below—indeed, nothing in all creation will ever be able to separate us from the love of God that is revealed in Christ Jesus our Lord." (Romans 8:38-39)
- "Now there is no condemnation for those who belong to Christ Jesus." (Romans 8:1)
- "See how very much our Father loves us, for he calls us his children, and that is what we are! But the people who belong to this world don't recognize that we are God's children because they don't know him." (1 John 3:1)
- "Let the Holy Spirit guide your lives. Then you won't be doing what your sinful nature craves." (Galatians 5:16)

PRAYER

....

Heavenly Father, in these weeks of the fast, we have focused on what we are eating, what spiritual disciplines we are practicing, and how this experience is affecting us. In all of these good things, please help us never to lose sight of the truth that You are already here and You are working! Thank You for the gift of the Holy Spirit, who is always with us. May we view this Daniel Fast not as a way to gain Your love, but as a way to experience more of You and Your love. As we deny ourselves this last week, show us how to turn to You and allow You to change us. May we grow ever closer to You as we learn to walk daily in the Spirit. Amen.

TIPS

- Keep reviewing your goals and your purpose for the fast each day. Don't give up! You're almost there.
- As you finish this week of the fast, continue to let your hunger pangs or cravings turn you toward God. I like to think of fasting as having a ribbon or rubber band fastened around my wrist to remind me to be purposeful in prayer and spiritual things.
- Let the Holy Spirit guide you about whether you should tell others that you are fasting. You don't want to call attention to yourself either through secrecy or by making a show of how much you're depriving yourself. Keep in mind, though, that others may be encouraged by knowing about your journey with fasting. If the Holy Spirit prompts you, be open to sharing your experience.
- If you are considering "pausing" the fast for a particular meal, think carefully about your motivation. Are you doing it for your own convenience? If so, I encourage you to remain steadfast and find a way to keep the fast you have committed to. However, if you want to "pause" out of love for someone else—for example, if friends have invited you to their home and prepared a meal especially for you—ask the Holy Spirit for guidance. If you do take a break from the fast, try to make it as brief as possible and then return to your usual routine.

- Remember, fasting and prayer are not ways to make God pay closer attention to us or tools we use to lobby Him and get Him to do what we want. God wants what is best for us already! He longs for us to be whole and healed and to experience more of His love and forgiveness. Pray this week for God's will to be done on earth and in your life.

Looking Forward after the Daniel Fast

REREAD IN *The Daniel Fast*:

- Pages 94–95 in Chapter 5 ("Five Steps for a Successful Daniel Fast")

GETTING STARTED

- How do you feel about your Daniel Fast concluding?

- What physical, mental, or spiritual surprises did you encounter during your Daniel Fast?

- What habits from your fasting experience do you want to carry forward in your everyday life?

- How has your experience changed your perspective on fasting?

- Reflect on the goals and purpose you set for your fast. How well do you think you achieved them? What can you do going forward to continue to work toward those goals?

CORE TRUTHS: LOOKING FORWARD

Over these past weeks, you have experienced something powerful. You have taken on a significant challenge, and you can feel good about persevering to the end. As you look back, remember that "finishing well" doesn't necessarily mean that you did everything perfectly, going all twenty-one days without a single food slipup and enjoying constant spiritual highs. Rather, it means that you stuck with what you had committed to do, even when it was tough. If you made a mistake or cheated, you admitted it, picked yourself back up, and tried again. You spent regular time with the Lord and found it rewarding, even if on some days it felt like you were going through the motions. You were open to the Holy Spirit's direction and saw Him working in your life. Finishing well means that you came through the twenty-one days changed in some way.

Now is the time to reflect back on your experience. This week you will consider these questions:

- What have you learned over these past weeks—about God or about yourself?

- How has the fast helped to renew your body, train your soul, and strengthen your spirit?

- How can you apply these lessons to your everyday life as you move forward?

SETTING THE SCENE

Read Ephesians 3:1-21.

When I think of all this, I, Paul, a prisoner of Christ Jesus for the benefit of you Gentiles . . . ²assuming, by the way, that you know God gave me the special responsibility of extending his grace to you Gentiles. ³As I briefly wrote earlier, God himself revealed his mysterious plan to me. ⁴As you read what I have written, you will understand my insight into this plan regarding Christ. ⁵God did not reveal it to previous generations, but now by his Spirit he has revealed it to his holy apostles and prophets.

⁶And this is God's plan: Both Gentiles and Jews who believe the Good News share equally in the riches inherited by God's children. Both are part of the same body, and both enjoy the promise of blessings because they belong to Christ Jesus. ⁷By God's grace and mighty power, I have been given the privilege of serving him by spreading this Good News.

⁸Though I am the least deserving of all God's people, he graciously gave me the privilege of telling the Gentiles about the endless treasures available to them in Christ. ⁹I was chosen to explain to everyone this mysterious plan that God, the Creator of all things, had kept secret from the beginning.

¹⁰God's purpose in all this was to use the church to display his wisdom in its rich variety to all the unseen rulers and authorities in the heavenly places. ¹¹This was his eternal plan, which he carried out through Christ Jesus our Lord.

¹²Because of Christ and our faith in him, we can now come boldly and confidently into God's presence. ¹³So please don't lose heart because of my trials here. I am suffering for you, so you should feel honored.

¹⁴When I think of all this, I fall to my knees and pray to the Father, ¹⁵the Creator of everything in heaven and on earth. ¹⁶I pray that from his glorious, unlimited resources he will empower you with inner strength through his Spirit. ¹⁷Then Christ will make his home in your hearts as you trust in him. Your roots will grow down into God's love and keep you strong. ¹⁸And may you have the power to understand, as all God's people should, how wide, how long, how high, and how deep his love is. ¹⁹ *May you experience the love of Christ, though it is too great to understand fully. Then you will be made complete with all the fullness of life and power that comes from God.*

²⁰ *Now all glory to God, who is able, through his mighty power at work within us, to accomplish infinitely more than we might ask or think.* ²¹ *Glory to him in the church and in Christ Jesus through all generations forever and ever! Amen.*

1. What can we do to have our "roots . . . grow down into God's love" (verse 17)? In what ways did the Daniel Fast help you put down those roots?

2. Look through the passage and identify things that God will give to His children. What do these reveal about the way God views us and the love He has for us? Is that the way you typically think about God?

3. Look at Paul's prayer for the believers (verses 14-19). What are some of the things he asks for them? How do these differ from the requests in your typical prayers? How might your life be changed if you prayed Paul's prayer for yourself and your family?

4. Verse 20 reminds us that God is able to accomplish more than we can even ask or think. Take a moment to identify areas in your life where you are struggling. Ask God to work His will in those areas in a powerful way. Trust that nothing is too hard for Him!

POINT TO PONDER
....

"During your fast you have learned empowering lessons about living by faith and walking in the Spirit. As you move into your normal way of life, bring with it the lessons you've learned. Create a 'new normal' with your increased spiritual awareness, your new habits of consistently spending time in prayer and study, and the healthy dietary choices you've learned." (*The Daniel Fast*, Chapter 5)

DIGGING IN
....

This passage from Ephesians reminds us of how much God has for us. He calls us His children, He provides a lavish inheritance for us, and He allows us to come boldly into His presence. He is not a taskmaster we must win over through our good deeds. He is a loving Father who wants to bless us with spiritual riches. He has "endless treasures" available to us in Christ! Yet so often we settle for less—praying only for small, day-to-day items that will make our lives more comfortable—when we could be praying for inner strength through the Spirit, the glorious riches of Christ, and the power to understand God's amazing, life-transforming love.

Paul says that God's love is "wide" (touching the breadth of our experiences); "long" (extending all of our days); "high" (stretching to the heights of our good times); and "deep" (reaching to the depths of our struggles and despair). His love encompasses our whole being—body, soul, and spirit. He gives our bodies dignity by making them His dwelling place. He created us as individuals yet lovingly teaches us that our souls—the center of our human individuality—should not be in control of our lives. He made us spirits so that we might live forever with Him, and He shows us the great joy that can come by walking with the Holy Spirit. He loves us enough to call us away from what is easy and into situations where we must depend on Him.

In these three weeks of the Daniel Fast, getting out of your usual routine and focusing on your relationship with God may have given you a glimpse of the "something more" that He has for you. Don't be satisfied with getting a taste of God and then returning to your old life. Pray for the courage to be changed and renewed by our life-giving Father.

DISCOVERING AND DOING

Your Daniel Fast lasted twenty-one days, and now it's over. In many ways, your experience was similar to that of a long-distance runner. You completed the "race" and now feel a sense of accomplishment and satisfaction. You're done! You made it!

As we discussed earlier, however, this should not simply be the end, but also the beginning (or a continuation) of living out those spiritual lessons and disciplines you learned during the fast. Growing in faith is a continuous, lifelong process—like putting down your roots to draw nourishment—not a onetime or short-term event.

Maybe God has gotten your attention through the Daniel Fast, and now He has more that He wants to teach you. For many people, fasting is a way to energize their relationships with God. It gets us out of our ruts and routines and challenges us to experience Him in a new way. The Daniel Fast can be a powerful three weeks—but its impact, if we let it, can last much longer. Consider these questions as you move into the post-fast period:

1. How will you remain attentive to God's voice in your life? What spiritual disciplines will you keep in place to help you find times to be quiet before God, listening to His direction?

2. When you don't have fasting to constantly help turn your mind toward God, how will you maintain a sense of His presence? Perhaps you can identify something else that will serve as a trigger for you to remember that God is with you and that He is part of every aspect of your life.

3. What new insights did you gain about the character of God and your identity in Him? How can these affect your life going forward?

4. What Scripture passages were important to you during your fast? Identify a few and consider committing them to memory.

5. Think carefully about when you might consider fasting again.

PRAYER

Heavenly Father, as we look back on these past three weeks, we are filled with gratitude. Thank You for meeting us in our fasting experience. Thank You for challenging us to develop self-discipline and to set our thoughts on You. We are grateful for all the ways You have been working in our lives over the past twenty-one days and for the ways You will continue to work. Please don't let the benefits from this experience slip away, but give us the perseverance to continue making our relationship with You the most important thing in our lives. Thank You for Your immeasurable love for us, Your children. In Jesus' name, Amen.

TIPS

Getting ready for your Daniel Fast required a significant amount of preparation as you anticipated three weeks of eating very differently than usual. I encourage you to plan for the end of your fast in a similar way. Your body, soul, and spirit have all experienced a great deal of change, and it's helpful to consider these changes carefully before you revert to old habits.

- How have you felt physically on the Daniel Fast? Many people experience increased energy and better health while they are fasting. Perhaps you have made a good start on breaking an addiction to sugar or certain junk foods. Think about whether you should continue to avoid those foods even when you're finished with the fast. If you decide to return to eating them, consider consuming them in smaller quantities and less frequently than before. Similarly, if you have gained good habits of healthy eating—such as consuming more fruits and vegetables—make a plan to help you continue these new patterns.
- If you reintroduce caffeine, sugar, dairy products, deep-fried foods, and meat to your diet, do it slowly to keep your body from rebelling and bringing you discomfort. Eat small portions at first, and try to add only one type of food each day to give your body a chance to get used to the change.
- Continue to drink at least sixty-four ounces of filtered water each day.
- As you reflect on the spiritual understanding you gained through the fast, consider how you can continue to grow. For example, if you have developed a habit of meeting with the Lord each morning or if you have experienced a new excitement about studying the Scriptures, keep it up! Carry these positive changes into your everyday life.
- It is common for people to feel let down at the end of their fast. If you have experienced a spiritual high, it's

understandable that going back to "normal life" will seem unexciting. But you don't have to go back to the way things were! Take some time to journal about the things you felt God teaching you throughout the fast. What might your next step be? How can you extend what you have learned about your body, soul, and spirit?

- Let the lessons you learned during your Daniel Fast continue to bring more health to your body, soul, and spirit all year long.

Leader's Guide

··

THANK YOU for being willing to serve in leading a group through the Daniel Fast. You are about to embark on a powerful experience that will bring you closer to God in a new way. It is my prayer that as you guide others through this fast, you and your group will be blessed richly.

As you read through the material in these pages, keep in mind that this is merely a *guide*. You know your group better than anyone, so you should feel free to adapt the questions to the needs of the group, members' personalities, and your leadership style. Be sure to keep in mind the objective for each lesson (spelled out in each session's "Core Truths" section), and then move the discussion toward meeting that goal.

PURPOSE

The ultimate purpose of these lessons is to deepen each participant's personal relationship with God. Completing the Daniel Fast, reading *The Daniel Fast* (including the Twenty-One-Day Daniel Fast Devotional), and participating in this group will move group members in that direction. It's also critical that they take time in Session 1 (the week of preparation) to think through their goals for the fast. This step is key in giving participants a sense of purpose that will motivate them to persevere to the end. Encourage everyone in your group to write down their goals and review them at least once a week.

LOGISTICS

- The study is intended to span five weeks. Week 1 will be preparation for the fast, Weeks 2–4 will encompass the three weeks of the fast, and Week 5 will be a session of reflection on what participants have experienced.
- On pages xvii–xviii we've indicated an approximate time range you might spend on each section of the lesson (assuming a 45–60 minute study).
- Ideally, participants should read through the lesson ahead of time and answer the questions on their own, then come together for discussion and support. As you prepare the material, you may want to highlight questions or sections you find most helpful. If your time is running short, focus on those areas.
- This study can work in a variety of formats, such as a small group, Sunday school class, or Bible study group. Of course, smaller groups will enable all the members to take an active

part in discussion. If your group is larger than a dozen people, consider dividing into smaller groups for at least part of the discussion (perhaps the "Getting Started" questions) to allow everyone to participate.

GETTING UP AND RUNNING

- Before you meet each week, ask God for His guidance as you lead the discussion. Pray that the conversation will be uplifting and that the participants will be spurred on to pursue greater intimacy with their Savior. In addition, ask God to help you discern who in the group needs special encouragement to continue with the fast, to do the assignments, and to go deeper in Bible study and prayer.
- As a fellow participant in the Daniel Fast, you will be able to identify with members' feelings and reflections. Be honest about your own experiences, both positive and negative. Know that your most important role as a group leader is to encourage those in your group to "fight the good fight" and continue in the fast, concentrating on the spiritual reasons for working toward this goal.
- Discuss with your group when you will start the Daniel Fast. It works best if everyone in the group begins the fast on the same day. However, this may not be possible because of differing schedules. Have a target start date and encourage your group members to begin as close to that day as possible—preferably within a two- or three-day span. That way your experiences will be similar as you meet together for weekly discussions.

- It is up to you to determine when your group will meet during the week. For example, Session 2 is designed to cover days 1–7 of the fast, so you do not necessarily have to meet at the very beginning on day 1. Find the time that works best for your group.
- Consider setting up "fasting buddies" within the group so pairs of people can provide accountability, prayer support, and encouragement for each other. Suggest that each pair pray for each other daily, check in with each other every few days, and give practical support as needed.
- Do your best to make sure everyone who attends your group has an opportunity to share. Be sensitive to the quieter members and try to make space for them to talk. If one or two group members are dominating the conversation, consider directing questions to others.
- Work to create a caring environment that is a safe place for participants to share their struggles. Do your best to keep the atmosphere positive and uplifting rather than critical. Group members should strive to support each other through doubts and mistakes, always being mindful of the higher purpose behind the fast.
- Make sure all group members can articulate their purpose for fasting as well as their goals for the Daniel Fast. Come back to these each week to encourage participants to maintain the right focus.
- Uphold group members in prayer during the week, and encourage them to pray for each other too. Consider sharing prayer requests via text message or e-mail.

- It is likely that group members will approach you with questions about whether specific foods are permissible on the fast. Keep a copy of *The Daniel Fast* on hand to help you respond to those questions, and encourage members to look at the blog and FAQ on www.daniel-fast.com. Remind group members to read the ingredient labels on all prepared foods.
- Many Bible study groups or small groups are accustomed to serving food at their meetings. Discuss with your group whether or not you will do this. If you will, make sure water is the only beverage available and that all food served is permissible on the fast. For ideas, look at the snack recipes included in *The Daniel Fast*. Also, avoid the temptation to overeat or include a lot of "forbidden" foods at the final meeting. Remember, it's important, for health reasons, to break the fast gradually.

HANDLING TOUGH ISSUES

Every group environment has a few tricky interactions:

- **Slipping up on the fast.** In a group of people doing the Daniel Fast, it is likely that at least one person will eat a food that is not allowed. If this is accidental, gently point it out and encourage the person to get back on track. However, things get trickier if people choose to ignore certain restrictions of the fast (not for medical reasons) and are unwilling to change. If this happens, extend grace and encourage all the group members to stick with their commitments. Use this as an opportunity to help people see that they are allowing their flesh to control their choices.

- **Dropping out.** A similar question is whether someone can remain in the group if he or she has stopped participating in the fast. Again, I encourage you to ask for the Holy Spirit's guidance for your particular situation. Generally, I feel that someone who is no longer fasting *may* remain in the group as long as he or she is sensitive to those who are still fasting and is not overly vocal about quitting. That person can still be an encouragement to those who are fasting and perhaps may grow to understand the factors that made the fast so difficult—or even be inspired to try fasting again later.
- **Wrong motivations.** You may have some group members who seem to be fasting for all the wrong reasons. If people in your group express that they're fasting solely to lose weight, for example, you will need to gently remind them that the point of the Daniel Fast is to limit certain foods *for a spiritual purpose.* Encourage them to develop their own spiritual goals for the fast. Likewise, if others seem to be fasting in an attempt to win God's approval, reassure them with the knowledge that they are God's children and are already greatly loved by Him. Remind them that the fast is a way for them to draw closer to God and learn to walk in the Spirit—not a way to find favor with Him.
- **"Pausing" from the fast.** If a group member wants to "pause" the fast for a particular reason, don't feel that you must be the "fasting police." This is between that person and the Holy Spirit. However, feel free to encourage all group members to seek the Spirit's guidance and to be aware of what might be motivating them to want to break the fast.

Your group members may encounter some challenges during their fasting experience. Your loving response to them is a central component to their success.

- **It's not about the food!** It's very easy for someone to make the fast all about the food and miss the powerful spiritual benefits of fasting. If you sense group members are talking too much about what they eat and cook and "can't have," turn the conversation into a teaching point. Perhaps you, too, have wrestled with this issue to "tell on yourself." Explain to the group how you realized that there is an internal battle going on between the spirit and the flesh and that when we spend so much time serving our flesh, we are "controlled by our sinful nature," as Paul describes in Romans 8:5-8 and 1 Corinthians 3:1-3.
- **Mistakes.** Group members may make a mistake or intentionally eat foods not allowed on the fast. First, they need not start over, just as we don't have to be "re-saved" if we go against God's ways. However, it's important to search our hearts and learn from the experience. Was the mistake made out of ignorance? If so, how can this be remedied on the fast (study, learn, prepare)? Ask members to consider other areas of their lives. Do they often enter into other situations unprepared? They don't need to answer in front of the group, but reflecting on the answer can be a powerful, life-changing experience for them. If someone has intentionally not followed the fasting guidelines, it's likely this might be a pattern that also appears in other settings—perhaps at work, at school, or in relationships. Help members see how these

issues during the fast are most likely a reflection of how we behave in our lives overall. Let's learn and grow and become better!

- **Emotional issues and deep wounding** can be uncovered during focused prayer and fasting. Don't feel that you need to *fix* these issues, but instead offer a road map for these participants by encouraging them to lift their needs to God, to find helpful study materials that can give them some solutions, and to meet with someone else in the church or community who could offer them appropriate help, if necessary. You may want to pray briefly about the matter and then move on so you can stay on track with the group meeting.

ADDITIONAL MATERIAL

Icebreaker Ideas

The questions in each week's "Getting Started" section should provide a good way to begin every discussion. However, if the participants in your group do not already know each other, you may want to use some neutral icebreaker questions in the first meeting to help build relationships. Here are a few suggestions:

- Where would you most like to travel?

- Tell us about one of your favorite holiday traditions.

- What was the last book you read, and what did you enjoy about it?

- Describe your favorite movie.

- If you had a day free from responsibilities, what would you do?

- What is one activity you look forward to every summer?

Questions for Further Discussion

If you find yourself with extra time in any given week, you may use any of these questions to foster discussion in your group:

- Which devotion resonated most with your fasting experience this week?

- What do you do when you're feeling discouraged on the fast?

- What is already working well in your fast? What's something you might change or do differently in the coming days?

- What recipes from the book have you tried and enjoyed?

- What has surprised you about the Daniel Fast?

May the five weeks of meeting together be filled with new insights and refreshing times with the Lord and with each other. Be blessed!

About the Author

Susan Gregory ("The Daniel Fast Blogger") regularly corresponds with thousands of men and women who are seeking God through the spiritual disciplines of prayer and fasting. Since its launch in December 2007, her site has received nearly nine million visits. Susan has written for nationally known preachers and ministries, including Charles Swindoll, Focus on the Family, Campus Crusade for Christ, and several third-world relief and development organizations. Her work has taken her to more than thirty-five countries. Susan is the author of *The Daniel Fast*, *Out of the Rat Race*, and *The Daniel Cure* (with Richard J. Bloomer, PhD). A mother and grandmother, she lives on a small farm in Central Washington. Visit her at www.daniel-fast.com.

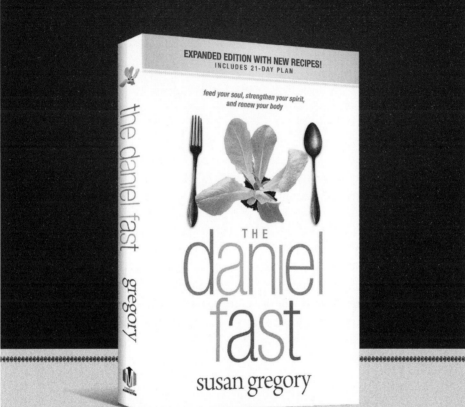

The Daniel Cure

The Daniel Fast Way to Vibrant Health

Susan Gregory, Author of Bestselling The Daniel Fast, and Richard J. Bloomer

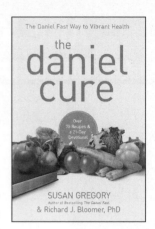

Though most people begin the Daniel Fast for a spiritual purpose, many are amazed by the physical transformation that takes place, such as a drop in cho-lesterol, healthy weight loss, a sense of well-being, and increased energy. Recently published scientific studies of the Daniel Fast documented many of the same findings, as well as a reduction in systemic inflammation and blood pressure, and improved antioxi-dant defenses. *The Daniel Cure* helps readers take the next step by focusing on the health benefits of the Daniel Fast. Following the advice in this book, readers will convert the Daniel Fast from a once-a-year spiritual discipline into a new way of life.

Includes a 21-Day Daniel Cure Devotional, frequently asked questions, ten chapters of recipes, a recipe index, and an appendix detailing "The Science behind the Daniel Fast."

Available in stores and online October 22, 2013!

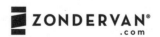

ZONDERVAN®
.com